FUNGAL NAIL INFECTION

GUIDE FOR TAKING CARE OF YOUR NAIL

TO PREVENT INFECTION

DR. DANNY JENSEN

Contents

CHAPTER ONE

Fungal nail contamination

Nail fungus is a commonplace contamination of the nail. It begins as a white or yellow-brown spot under the tip of your fingernail or toenail. Because the fungal infection goes deeper, the nail can also discolor, thicken and fall apart at the threshold. Nail fungus may have an impact on numerous nails.

If your situation is moderate and no longer bothering you, you may no longer want treatment. In case your nail fungus is painful and has brought on thickened nails, self-care steps and medicines may additionally moreover assist. But despite the fact that remedy is a hit, nail fungus regularly comes decrease again.

Nail fungus is also known as onychomycosis (on-ih-koh-my-KOH-sis). While fungus infects the regions among your feet and the skin of your ft, it's known as athlete's foot (tinea podis).

A fungal nail infection is a not unusual circumstance which can go away you with brittle, discolored nails, generally for your ft.

Its formal call is onychomycosis, and it's plenty like athlete's foot. However in desire to affecting the pores and skin on the bottom of your feet or between your ft, it invades your nails.

Fungi are tiny organisms you can fine see through a microscope. Many differing types can motive a nail contamination. Once in a while they stay on your pores and skin and don't make any hassle. However if you have lots in a unmarried vicinity, you can get inflamed.

Don't be embarrassed when you have toenail or fingernail fungus. It's manner more common than you believe you studied.

With toenail fungus, your nail turns into thick and yellow and can display white spots and streaks. A sort of mildew known as a dermatophyte causes tinea unguium, the maximum common nail fungus. Tinea unguium maximum regularly objectives your toenails, but it can also have an impact for your fingernails. Onychomycosis is another call for the circumstance.

Toenail fungus is a exquisite fungal contamination that influences your toenails. Lots much less normally, nail fungus can infect your fingernails. Toenail fungus takes area while fungi get amongst your toenail and your toenail bed (the tissue right under your toenail). This commonly takes location via a crack or cut in your toe.

Varieties of Fungal Nail Infections

There are 4 crucial styles of fungal nail infection. Every seems slightly one-of-a-type:

Distal or lateral subungual onychomycosis. This is the most not unusual kind. It results from a fungus known as a dermatophyte. You can get it to your fingernails or toenails.

It starts in the nail mattress, underneath the nail. You'll see a yellowish coloured location that spreads from the rims of the nail to the center, and locations wherein it comes aside from the nail bed.

White superficial onychomycosis. This is an awful lot less commonplace and most effective impacts the nail surface, specifically for your toenails. It begins as white spots, which become powdery and reason the nail to collapse.

Proximal subungual onychomycosis. This appears first as white spots in the center of the nail bed at the cuticle. They flow into outward because the finger or toenail grows. It's rare and typically influences human beings who have immune system troubles, like HIV infection.

Candidal onychomycosis. Yeast causes this infection that normally influences your fingernails. The area across the nails is regularly swollen and infected, and the nails may moreover come off absolutely. It has a tendency to appear to nails which have been broken by way of an damage or some other contamination.

What is tinea unguium?

While a dermatophyte reasons toenail fungus, the circumstance is called tinea unguium. A dermatophyte is a mold that dreams a protein referred to as keratin to develop. Keratin is the principle structural material of your nails that makes them tough. Dermatophytes cause 90% of toenail fungal infections. Tinea unguium is likewise called onychomycosis.

Who does toenail fungus affect?

Absolutely all of us can get toenail fungus. It often affects older adults, mainly people over 60.

You may have a better threat of having toenail fungus when you have:

Athlete's foot (tinea pedis).

Diabetes.

Hyperhidrosis (a sickness that makes you sweat a lot).

A nail harm.

Terrible blood motion due to peripheral vascular ailment.

Psoriasis.

A weakened immune device, together with from an autoimmune sickness or HIV.

Fungal Nail infection signs

Symptoms are first rate, relying on which kind of fungal nail contamination you have got. They usually start mild and get more crucial.

Earlier than the whole lot, you could handiest see a white or yellow spot beneath your nail. Over time, this spreads and can flip your whole nail white, yellow, green, or black.

The nail may thicken and is probably difficult to trim.

It may begin to curl up or down or loosen from the nail mattress.

Your nail ought to become brittle and crumble whilst you contact it.

Your nail may additionally additionally end up misshapen.

You may phrase a bad smell.

It's clean to brush aside fungal nail infections on the start, because of the fact you may now not have any pain. But in case you don't deal with them, it is able to damage to place any pressure on the area. If an contamination gets horrible enough, it is able to even grow to be difficult to walk.

CHAPTER TWO

What reasons tinea unguium?

A sort of mildew known as a dermatophyte causes tinea unguium. Dermatophytes are fungal microorganisms (too tiny to look with the naked eye). They feed off of keratin, a protein located in your fingernails and toenails. Keratin makes nails difficult.

Dermatophytes are the motive within the lower back of ninety% of toenail fungal infections. However other styles of fungi can infect your toenails as well.

Is tinea unguium contagious?

Sure, many types of toenail fungi, which encompass tinea unguium, are pretty contagious. You may spread the fungus to someone else through direct contact. You may additionally get toenail fungus with the aid of using touching an infected floor.

What are common strategies you can get toenail fungus?

Nail fungi like warm, moist, dark locations. You could get toenail fungus by using:

On foot across the perimeters of swimming swimming pools.

Using a public locker room or shower.

Strolling barefoot in a public place.

Can toenail fungus unfold to one-of-a-kind regions of your frame?

Sure. But toenail fungus generally doesn't unfold beyond your toe.

Some dermatophyte fungi spread effortlessly for your pores and pores and skin. (Your skin and scalp moreover contain keratin.) when dermatophyte fungi have an effect on your pores and pores and skin, the condition is referred to as ringworm.

Toenail fungus may additionally additionally spread to:

Other toenails.

Pores and pores and skin among your toes (known as athlete's foot).

Groin region (known as jock itch).

Scalp (pores and pores and skin on top of

your head).

While to peer a physician

You could want to look a health care agency if self-care steps have not helped and the nail turns into more and more discolored, thickened or misshapen. Moreover talk together with your fitness care company if you have:

Diabetes and assume you're growing nail fungus

Bleeding around the nails

Swelling or pain throughout the nails

Trouble taking walks

Threat elements

Factors which could boom your hazard of growing nail fungus include:

Older age

Sporting shoes that make your feet sweat intently

Having had athlete's foot in the beyond

Walking barefoot in damp public regions, consisting of swimming swimming swimming pools, gyms and bathe rooms

Having a minor pores and pores and skin or nail damage

Having a pores and skin situation that impacts the nails, together with psoriasis

Having diabetes, blood drift problems or a weakened immune machine

Headaches

A excessive case of nail fungus may be painful and might motive permanent damage to your nails. And it is able to bring about one of a kind crucial infections that spread beyond your feet when you have a suppressed immune device due to medicinal drug, diabetes or other situations.

Fungal Nail contamination treatment

See your doctor in case you assume you have got were given nail fungus. It can be tough to do away with, and also you're much more likely to have fulfillment with a prescription. Remedies encompass:

Oral antifungals. The medical doctor might also additionally give you a pill to kill fungus for your whole frame. That is generally the exceptional way to get rid of a nail infection. Remedy may last 2 months for an contamination on your fingernails, or 3 months if it's in your toenails.

Topical antifungals. You rub or brush those drug treatments onto your nails. They may paintings for a mild infection, but they can't get deep sufficient into the nail to remedy a greater extreme one. You can use a topical treatment in mixture with a tablet.

Surgical operation. If special remedies don't artwork, the doctor may also need to take away your nail completely and permit a healthful one broaden lower back in its place. The modern nail can also get infected.

Laser or photodynamic therapy. Doctors are

studying more recent remedies that use special moderate to try to kill the fungus.

How is toenail fungus diagnosed?

Your healthcare issuer will first look intently on the affected toenail to evaluate your signs and symptoms and signs and symptoms. They may be capable of understand toenail fungus virtually with the aid of searching at your toe. But, your corporation may also order assessments to confirm a fungal contamination.

What tests might be accomplished to diagnose toenail fungus?

Your healthcare provider will possibly take a small sample from under your nail to similarly study it. Viewing the cells underneath a microscope can confirm a toenail fungus diagnosis. If the initial take a look at is poor, a scraping can be despatched to look if the fungus grows out in a tradition. This additionally facilitates your healthcare provider discover the shape of fungus.

How am i able to save you toenail fungus?

There's no way to assure you gained't get toenail fungus. But you can take numerous steps to help prevent it:

Keep away from going barefoot in communal areas including public showers, locker rooms and swimming swimming pools. The general public select up fungus in the ones situations. It facilitates to put on flip flops in the ones public areas.

If you have a member of the family with foot fungus or nail fungus, try and use a special bathe or wear turn flops within the bathe to avoid coming in touch with it.

Trauma because of accidental or competitive clipping of the nails can emerge as portals of entry for the fungus.

Easy your nail trimmer earlier than using it.

Don't tear or rip your toenails on cause.

When you have diabetes, take a look at all foot care recommendations from your healthcare enterprise.

Maintain your toes dry. Make sure to completely dry your ft after a bath.

Soak toenails in heat water before slicing them. Or you may lessen your nails after a bathtub or bath.

Trim toenails at once in the course of (don't round the edges).

Placed on footwear that in form effectively. They shouldn't be too loose or tight across the toes.

What am i capable of count on if i've a toenail fungus?

Even as toenail fungus is commonplace, it's usually now not dangerous. Signs and symptoms within the principal have an impact on the arrival of your toenail.

Toenail fungus may moreover unfold to the pores and skin among your toes or one-of-a-kind areas of your body. Whilst getting dressed, placed your socks on first to reduce the threat of unfold.

Treating toenail fungus takes a long time, and it doesn't generally work. Even then, toenail fungus regularly returns. Communicate the pros and cons of treating toenail fungus together with your healthcare company to determine what's first-class for you.

Running toward particular hygiene and foot care reduces the threat toenail fungus will come lower back. When you have diabetes, getting normal foot tests may additionally moreover assist you cope with foot issues before they get critical.

Can i put on nail polish if i've toenail fungus?

You may experience tempted to cowl up a discolored toenail with nail polish. However in case you're using a topical antifungal, you possibly shouldn't use polish. Your healthcare provider may also assist you to recognise no longer to place on it anyhow.

Nail polish traps in moisture out of your nailbed (the tissue below your toenail). Due to the fact fungi thrive in moist environments, wearing nail polish also can make a fungal infection worse. However, your nail continues to increase without or with polish.

CONCLUSION

Toenail fungus (tinea unguium) is an exceptionally commonplace infection that can be difficult to cope with. Tinea unguium typically isn't painful, however it could make you experience self-aware of how your foot appears. If it bothers you, communicate on your healthcare company about your treatment options. A skilled specialist (which includes a dermatologist or podiatrist) can provide guidance on what's most in all likelihood to cope with your worries at the same time as protective your common health.

THE END